[

Workouts At Home For Women

The Best Exercises to Lose Weight Without Any Special Equipment

Table of Contents

Introduction

This book will help you stop worrying about finding that perfect gym, the right attire, the right equipment or finding the space or time to exercise. You are carefully choosing what to eat and what to avoid. However, you will feel much richer and happier if you were in better shape.

You don't have to spend money or find time to go to a gym to get fitter; the book will show you how to perform effective exercises that any beginner can do with only dumbbells or without any exercise equipment in the comfort of your own home. The book gives you 50 different exercises for your upper body, shoulders, arms, chest, back, lower body and legs. Start to practice these exercises, and within a month, your body will change from inside out.

Double Dumbbells Exercise

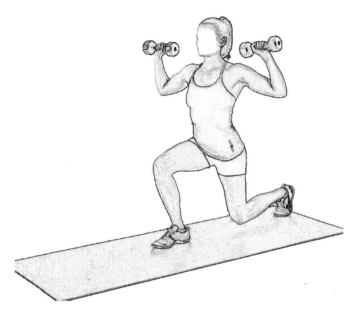

o Do some light cardio and warm up for five minutes.

o Then grab two sets of dumbbells between 5 to 25 pounds.

o Start with 10 reps of each exercise and gradually increase to 15 repetitions.

Plank and Rotate

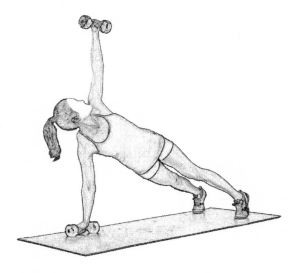

o   The exercise is best for the core muscles.

o   Start with a plank pose by holding a five-pound dumbbell in each hand. To protect your joints, keep your wrists stiff and spread your feet a little wider than your hip distance.

o   Twisting through your entire upper body, raise your left hand upward. Keep your pelvis level even though it will rotate.

o   Lower your hand toward the floor and repeat the exercise with your right hand.

o   Practice 10 to 15 times to complete a set.

Single-Leg Scarecrows

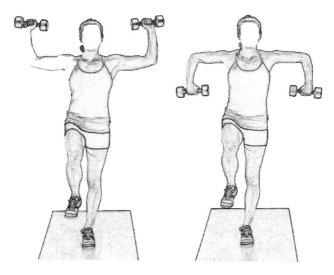

○   Begin by standing on your left leg. Then gradually raise your right knee upward until it is level with your hip. In your each hand, hold a dumbbell and lift the arms until your upper arms are parallel to the ground. Now bend the elbows 90 degrees.

○   Hold the pose steadily. Bring your fists to the floor by rotating your upper arms forward. Then bring the fists up by rotating the upper arm backward. Do not raise or lower your upper arms, keep them parallel to the floor. This will complete one rep.

○   Practice 10 to 15 times, then switch legs and practice with the other foot. Do 10 to 15 reps to complete the set.

Squat, Curl and Press

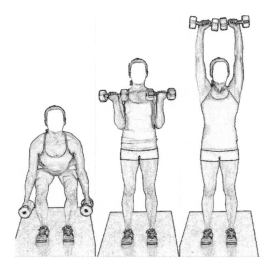

o   Holding a dumbbell in each hand, stand with your feet directly under your hips. Keeping the weight in your hands, sit back into your squat. Then without letting your knees go beyond your toes, bring your thighs parallel to the floor.

o   Press on your heels, get back up and perform a bicep curl by bringing the weights to your shoulders.

o   Steady your upper body and perform an overhead press by continue to lift your arms upward, keep your palms facing out.

o   Bring your arms back to your side to complete one rep.

o   Practice 10 to 15 reps.

Lying Chest Fly

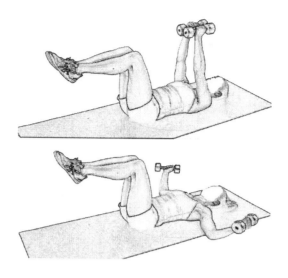

- ○ Lie on your back on the floor. Keep your knees and hips both at 90-degree angles. Press your lower back into the mat using your lower abs. Lift your arms upward, keep the elbow joint slightly bent and palms facing each other.

- ○ Steady your upper body, then continue to stretch your arms out to the side until your elbows are almost touching the floor.

- ○ Lift your arms back upward, bring the weight closer to your upper body. This complete one rep.

- ○ Do 15 reps to complete one set.

Lying Overhead Reach

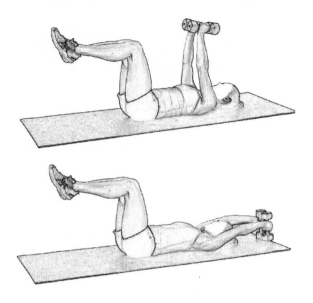

o Lie on your back on the floor, keep your knees and hips both at 90-degree angles. Use the low abs to push your lower back directly onto the mat. Lift your arms upward and keep your elbow joint bent slightly.

o Lift your arms over your head, and move the dumbbells to tap the dumbbells on the floor above your head. As you lower the weights, don't allow your back arch away from the floor.

o Shift your hands to the starting position to complete one rep.

o Do 15 reps to complete a set.

Seated Russian Twist

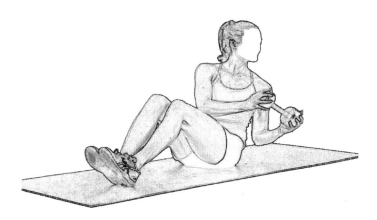

o   Sit on the floor and keep your heels about two feet away from your butt while holding a dumbbell at your chest. Lean your entire upper body back a few inches while keeping your back straight. The pose should make you feel like your abs are trying to keep your body upright.

o   Rotate your ribcage to the left, without rounding your spine, then return to the center to twist to the right. You have finished one rep.

o   Do 15 reps to complete a set.

Reverse Lunge and Press

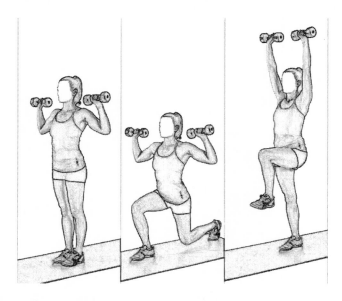

o Stand straight while holding the weight on your shoulders. Palm facing out and feet together.

o Step the left foot backward coming into a lunge, making 90-degree angles with your back and front knee.

o Bring your left knee forward while pushing off your left foot. So it is parallel with your left hip while raising the arms upward. Steady yourself and then do it.

o Step back into the lunge without touching the floor with your left foot and start the second rep.

o Do 15 reps, then switch legs.

Plank and Straight-Arm Kickback

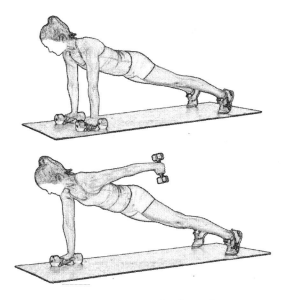

o Holding a dumbbell in each hand, start in a plank position. For a stronger base of support, open your feet wider than hip width.

o Raise your left arm as high as you can behind you. Complete one rep by bringing the left arm back into plank.

o Do 10 to 15 reps with each arm.

Weighted Squat

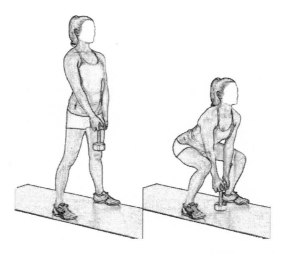

o   Holding one dumbbell in both hands, stand and keep your feet a little wider than your hips, toes facing slightly outward.

o   Keeping the weight in your chest and heels lifted; sit back to squat. The dumbbell bottoms should slightly touch the floor.

o   Push through the heels to go back to standing position to complete one rep.

o   Do 15 reps.

Upper Body: Push-Up

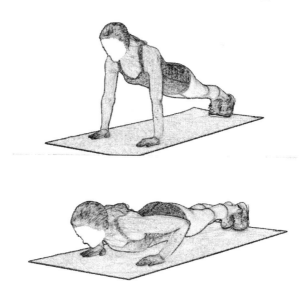

- ○ Start in a plank position, with your legs out behind you, shoulders over your wrists and palms spread out evenly. Keep your back straight and pull your belly button in.

- ○ Bend your elbows outward to the sides, as you go lower and breathe out. Hold at the bottom before you get back up to finish one rep.

Upper Body: Diamond Push-Ups

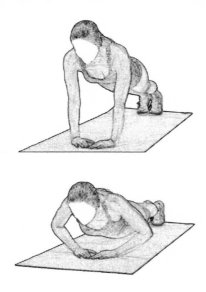

o   Start in plank position with your body in one straight line and your hands under your shoulders.

o   To help you stay balanced throughout the exercise, separate your feet to about shoulder-width apart.

o   Directly under your sternum, place your hands together, with the tips of your thumbs and fingers touching. Your thumbs and fingers should form a triangle or diamond shape.

o   As you lower your chest toward the floor, bend your elbows out to the sides. Then breathe out to straighten your arms. This completes one rep.

Upper Body: Superwoman

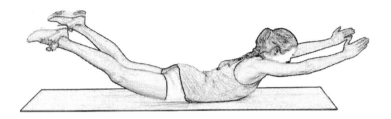

o   Lie on your belly on the floor. Engaging your abs spread your arms straight in front of you.

o   Raise your arms, chest, and legs off the floor. Hold the pose and count to 10, then gently release your body and go back to the floor. This finishes one rep.

Upper Body and Core: Plank Up and Down

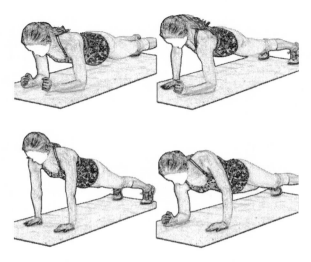

o   Go to a plank position with your legs and arms straight. Keep your feet hips-width distance apart and your hands underneath your shoulders.

o   Keeping your upper body parallel to the floor, lower your right forearm to the floor and come into elbow plank by lowering the left.

o   Then push yourself back up to plank position by step the right hand back onto the mat, and then the left. This completes one push-up walk.

Upper Body and Core: Lateral Plank Walk

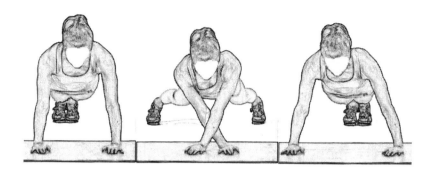

o   Start in plank position with your body in one straight line and your hands underneath your shoulders.

o   As you step your left foot out to the left, simultaneously cross your right hand toward the left. Then return to the plank position by simultaneously stepping your right foot and left hand to the left. As your feet step apart, your hands move together. Keeping your pelvis level and abs pulled toward your spine; take two more steps in this direction. This finishes one rep.

o   Take three steps to the right and reverse directions.

Upper Body and Core: Push-Up and Rotate

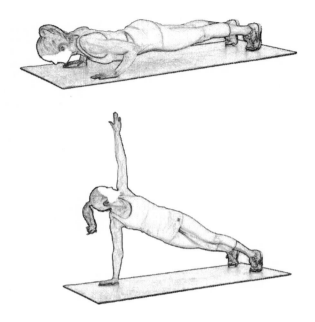

o   Start in a plank position with your hips and feet in a parallel position.

o   Gradually lower your body to the floor, then lift through your arms to go back to plank.

o   Twist to the left, then lift your arm toward the ceiling without allowing your pelvis go lower or raised.

o   Go back to the plank pose, and lower your head toward the floor. This will finish one rep.

Reverse Plank Bridge

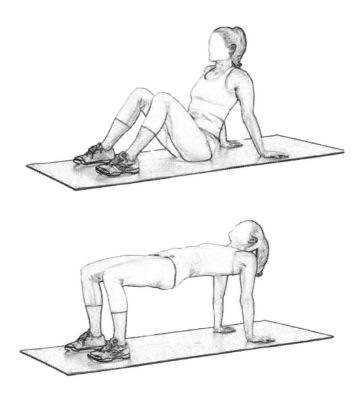

o   Start by sitting; keep your hands behind your body and fingers facing outward.

o   Raise your pelvis off the floor by pressing your hands and heels of your feet into the ground. Continue to raise until it is in line your knees and shoulders.

o   Bring your pelvis down to the ground to complete one rep.

Core: Bicycle Crunches

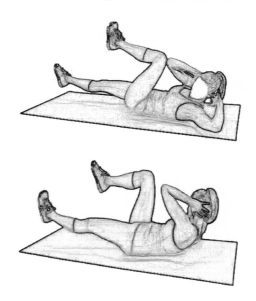

o   With your lower back pressed to the ground, lie flat on the ground. Put your hands behind your head and interlace your fingers.

o   Move your knees inward, close to your chest. Then raise your shoulder blades off the ground.

o   While turning your upper body to the left, straighten out the right leg to about a 45-degree angle to the ground and bring your right elbow toward the left knee. Remember both your elbows and rib cage need to be moved.

o   Now repeat with the other side of your body to complete one rep.

Core: Seated Russian Twist

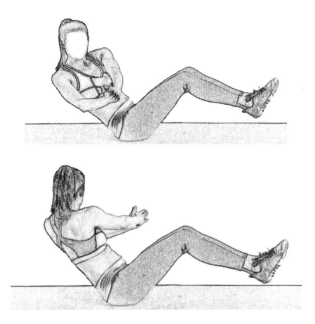

- o   With your knees bent, sit on the ground. Push your abs toward the spine and while lifting your feet off the floor, lean back a few inches. Keep your back straight.

- o   Meet your arms in front of your body and then twist your upper body to the right, then to the left. Continue for 1 minute. If you feel the need, lower your heels to the ground.

Core: Reverse Crunch

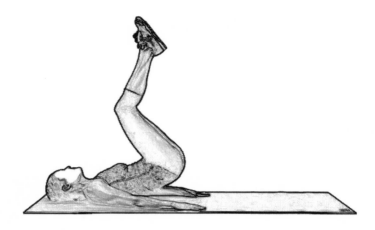

○ Lie back on your back and keep your hands beside your body.

○ Keep your feet together and bring your knees in toward your chest.

○ Slowly curl the hips off the floor and into your chest by using your abs. Then gradually lower them back to the beginning position to complete one rep.

○ Repeat for one minute. Use your abs to control your movement and don't swing your legs to create momentum.

Core: V-Sits

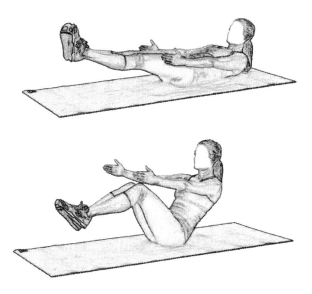

o   Lie on your back on the floor. Then reach the arms firmly beside your body, above the floor. Raise your legs off the floor and point them to about a 45-degree angle. Make sure your shoulders are off the floor by raising your hand.

o   Once you are ready to start, raise your upper chest off the floor, then bend the knees. Come up more to make this easier or lean back to make this move harder. If you choose easier, then gradually straighten out your legs and lower your chest back down to the floor. Stop once your back reaches the floor, but not your legs, shoulders or head.

o   This finishes one rep.

Core: Mountain Climbers

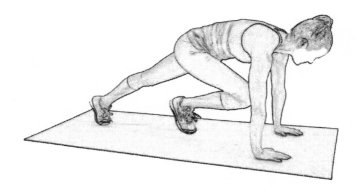

o To start go to a standard push-up starting position –
   weight on just on your toes and shoulders over your
   hands.

o Move the right foot forward, bending your knee and
   keeping your weight on the ball of your foot.

o Shift legs, while moving the right leg back, bring the left
   knee forward. You have finished one rep.

Core: Side Plank

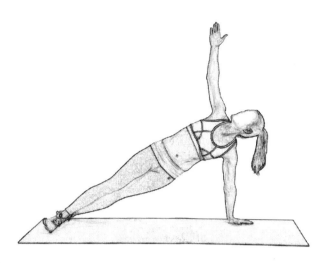

- ○ Sit on your left side with your feet stacked and legs slightly bent.

- ○ Position your left hand about 12 inches from the pelvis.

- ○ Press your hand into the ground. As you lift your pelvis off the ground, straighten your legs. The top leg should be in front, so stagger your feet if you have trouble balancing.

- ○ Hold the pose for 30 seconds, then switch sides to complete one rep.

Core: Full Sit-Ups

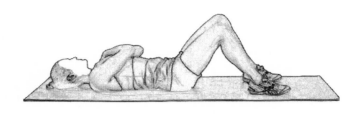

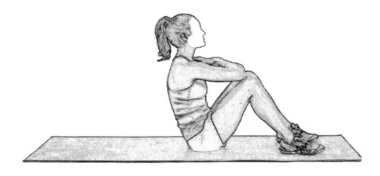

○ Lay on your back with your feet flat on the ground and knees bent. Position your hands on opposite shoulders.

○ Engage your abdominal muscles while keeping your toes flat on the ground and heels on the ground. Gradually lift your head first, then shoulder blades, go to a full sit-up position.

○ Hold the pose for a moment or two, then steadily come slowly back down to the floor.

○ This completes one full sit-up.

Lower Body: Good Morning

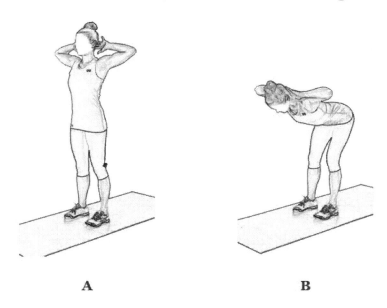

A   B

○   Stand straight and keep your feet hip-width apart. With your elbows opened wide, place your hands on the back of your head.

○   Pull your abs toward the spine. Keep your back neutral and hinging at the hips, press your butt backward, until your back is virtually analogous to the floor.

○   Go back the starting position. When you are upright, squeeze your glutes. This completes one rep.

Lower Body: Basic Squat

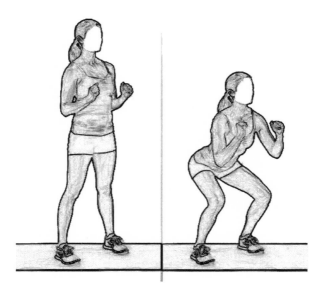

o   Stand straight and keep your feet shoulder-width apart.
    To help you stay balanced, hold your hands comfortably
    in front of your chest. Bend the knees and lower your
    hips deeply, so the thighs are analogous with the floor.
    Keep your weight back on the heels.

o   Now lift up. Squeezing the glutes at the top of the
    movement and straightening the legs completely to get
    the most out of the exercise.

o   You have finished one rep.

Lower Body: Wall Sit

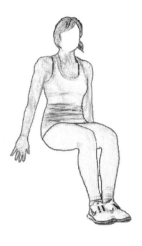

o   Placing your feet two feet in front of you, stand with your back against a wall. Keep your feet about hip-distance apart.

o   Gradually bend your knees and slide the back down the wall until you make a 90-degree angle with your knees. You may need to inch your feet further from the wall, so your knee joints are over your ankle joints and create a proper alignment. Don't allow your knees to sway outward or fall into the midline of your body.

Lower Body: Sumo Squat

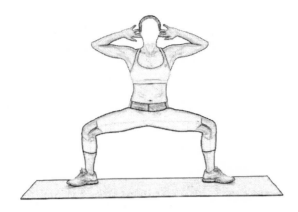

o   To start: stand and keep your legs wide and toes pointed marginally outward. With elbows wide, place your hands at your head to challenge your abs as you practice.

o   Continue to bend your knees until they are over your ankles. Your feet should be far enough apart that your knees near 90 degrees and thighs are parallel to the floor. Straighten your legs by a push through your heels.

o   This finishes one rep.

Lower Body: Side Lunge

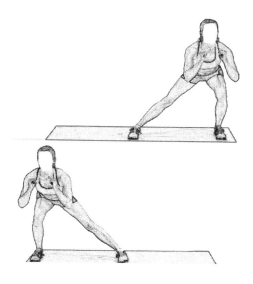

- Make 90-degree angles with both knees by going one step back with your left foot and go into a deep lunge.

- Continue to lift your arms outward away from your body until your upper arms analogous to the floor. Bend the elbows to 90 degrees and make flexible fists with your hands.

- Continue to hold the pose while you bring your fists to the floor by rotating your upper arms forward. Then rotate the upper arm backward to raise the fists. Do not raise or lower your upper arms, continue to keep them analogous to the floor.

- You have completed one rep.

Lower Body: Lunge

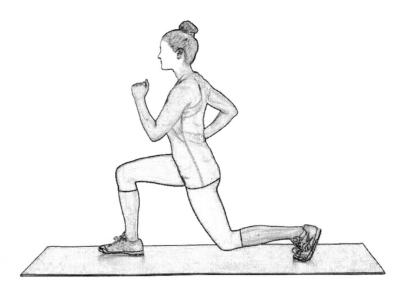

o   Keep your upper body straight, keep your chin up, and shoulders back and relaxed. Engage your core.

o   Step forward with one leg. Continue to lower your hips until your both knees are bent and create a 90-degree angle. Make sure your front knee is not pushed too far, and it is directly above your ankle. Your other knee must not touch the floor. Push back up to the starting position while keeping your weight on your heels.

o   You finished one lunge.

Lower Body: Single-Leg Balance Touch

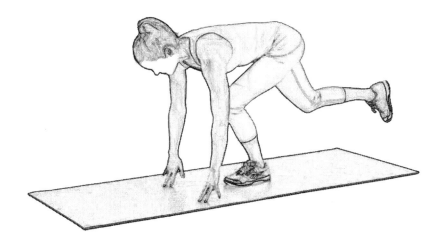

○   Start standing with all your weight on your left foot and your arms overhead.

○   Bending your left knee, touch both hands to the ground while keeping your spine long, reach forward. Keep your torso stable by keeping your abs engaged.

○   While lifting your torso, lower your right leg down. Bring the arms overhead to complete one rep.

Plyometrics: Jump Squat

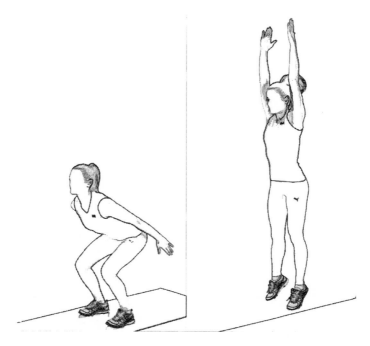

- With your arms by your sides, come up into a squat.

- As you jump off with both feet, swing your arms to the ceiling.

- Land quietly as you go back to the squat position.

- This finishes one rep.

Plyometrics: High-Knee Skips

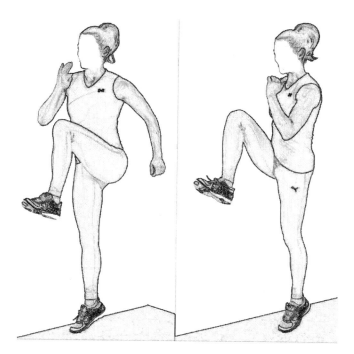

- By hopping on your right leg, skip in place while moving your left knee up toward your chest.

- As your knee comes toward your chest, engage your abs.

- Switch legs and continue to skip while pumping the arms.

- You completed one rep.

Standing Chop

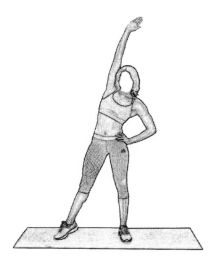

o   Stand with your feet hip-width apart.

o   While your right hand is resting on your hip, extend your left arm overhead.

o   Keeping your left knee flexible, bring your right knee upward and in a controlled chopping motion, pull the left arm down.

o   For one count, aim for the outside of your knee with your elbow.

o   Go back to the starting position.

o   Practice 8 to 10 times on each side of your body.

Criss-Cross

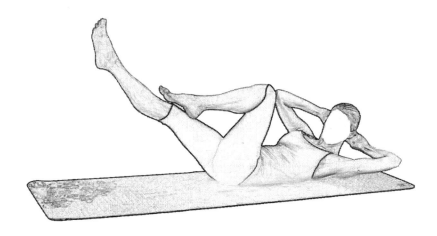

○ Lie down on your back. Slightly raise the top of your shoulder blades off the floor and clasp your hands behind your head.

○ As you twist at your waist, straighten and lift left leg off the floor.

○ Slowly bring your right knee in toward your left shoulder.

○ Hold the position for two counts, then twist to the opposite side of your body for one repetition.

○ Do 10 to 12 repetitions.

Hip Raise

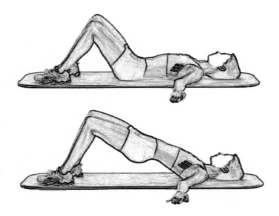

o   Lie down on your back with your feet flat on the floor, and knees bent.

o   At a 45-degree angle, place your arms out to your sides, with palms facing up.

o   While breathing normally, try to make your tummy as skinny as possible. Hold that position and continue to breathe normally.

o   Squeeze your glutes while keeping your core tight. Then lift your hips, so your body makes a straight line from your knees to your shoulders.

o   Squeezing your glutes tightly, pause for 5 seconds. Then return to the starting position.

o   Practice for 10 repetitions.

Side-Kick Plie

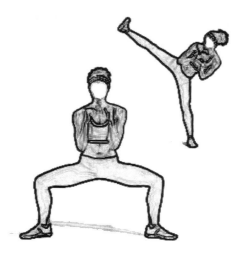

- ○ Stand straight and keep your feet two to three feet apart, toes turned outward.

- ○ Go to a squat position with fists in front of your chest and elbows bent.

- ○ Stand up and then lift your right leg off the floor.

- ○ Concentrate on your glutes, lower your left shoulder and kick your right leg outward.

- ○ Reverse the exercise to return to the previous squat position. You have finished one rep.

- ○ Do 10 and then repeat with your left leg.

AB Roll-Up

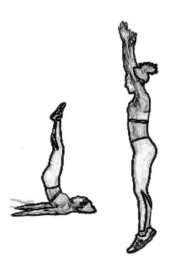

o   Sit on the floor and spread your legs in front of you. Roll your back onto the floor, then supporting your body with your arms; lift your legs over your hips.

o   Use this shifting movement to roll back to the beginning position, but place your feet flat on the floor and bend your knees.

o   Firmly place your feet and then jump upward and reaching your arms over the head.

o   Land gently and bend your knees to lower back down to start.

o   You have finished one rep. practice 10.

Standing Mountain Climber

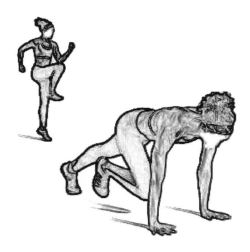

o   Jog for 10 counts to add a cardio component.

o   Bring your knees upward to your hip level.

o   Get into a plank position by dropping to the floor.

o   Then quickly alternate moving your knees to your chest 10 times.

o   You have completed one rep. jump up to and go back to the starting position.

o   Repeat three times.

L Stand

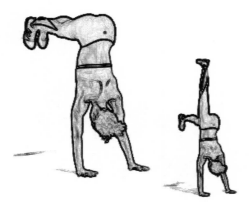

- o Against the bottom of a wall, place your heels. Then bend forward, and place your hands on the floor, keep them shoulder-width apart.

- o Walk your feet up the wall until your body forms a 90-degree angle, and your legs are parallel to the floor. This exercise works your shoulders and upper backs.

- o Activate your core by raising your right leg. Reverse to return to start.

- o This is one rep, practice 10 rep.

Bend and Thrust

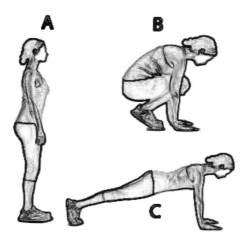

o   Stand straight.

o   Keep your feet hip-width apart and arms at your sides.

o   Bend the knees and on either side of your legs, position
    your hands on the floor, do it in one motion.

o   Now jump both feet back, so your body gets into a
    pushup position while you keep your back straight.

o   Quickly reverse the motion and go back to the starting
    position.

o   This is one rep.

Power Push-Offs

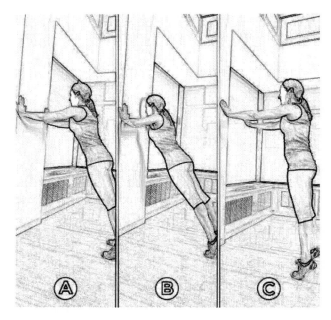

o   Place your hands on the wall. Keep them a little wider than shoulder-width apart and form a solid plank by step your feet back.

o   Bring your chest close to the wall by bending your elbows, then suddenly push back, so you tilt back on your toes, and your hands come off the wall.

o   Bending your arms, fall back into the wall. Do 8 rep.

Marching Bridges

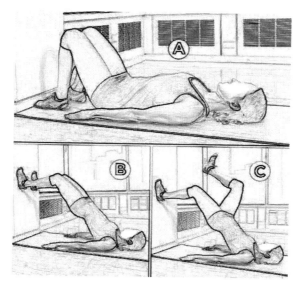

o Lie down on your back, with toes touching the wall; knees bent up and arms by your side.

o Walk your feet up the wall one-step. Make sure your body is flat from your knees to shoulders by pushing your hips.

o To keep your hips high, gradually move the legs closer to your chest at the same time associating your glute muscles.

o You need to exercise your both legs to complete one rep.

o Practice 8 reps.

L-Handstand Step-Ups

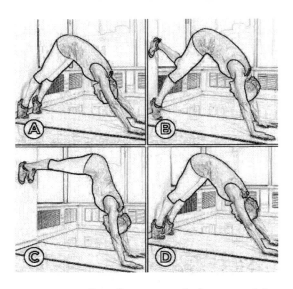

o   To start, go to the downward dog position while your heels touch the wall.

o   Raise one leg and place your foot on the wall about hip height.

o   With your raised foot, press into the wall and then raise your other foot and place it beside the first one.

o   In this modified handstand, pause briefly. Then step back down.

o   Start with one foot and practice 4 reps, then repeat reverse.

Foot-Up Split Squats

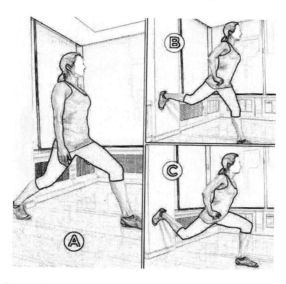

o Stand straight and keep your back toward the wall.
   Then take a large step forward.

o Raise your back leg and position your toe against the
   wall.

o Lean your upper body forward slightly by squaring off
   your hips.

o Gradually bend the front leg and continue to bend as
   long as you feel comfortable.

o Go back to straight position.

o Practice 8 reps on each leg.

Triceps Extension

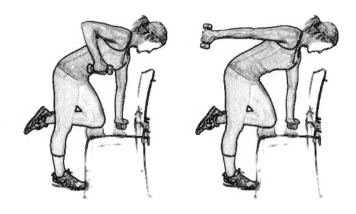

o   With your back heel on the ground, go into a lunge
    position.

o   As you lift your arm straight up by your side, lean over
    your bent front knee – keep the top of the weight facing
    upward.

o   Raise and then lower the weight about 1-inch 30 times
    to finish one rep.

Arnold Press

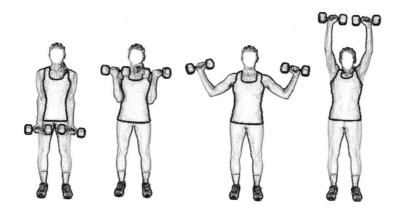

- ○ This classic exercise beneficial for the entire upper body, particularly for the shoulders

- ○ Grab the dumbbells; keep your elbows fixed and palms facing your body.

- ○ Extend your elbows and raise the dumbbells. Then bring your shoulders to a straight-arm position by internally rotating them.

- ○ Go back to original position and repeat.

Ball Crunch

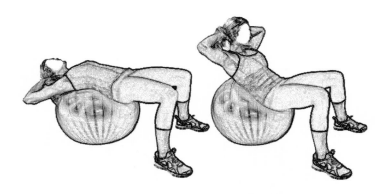

o Calmly sit on the exercise ball and move your legs
   forward to roll back onto the ball. Once you are settled,
   keep your spine in neutral alignment, position your
   hands behind the head, and slightly lift your chin
   toward the sky.

o Breathe out as you crunch up and breathe in as you
   release back down.

o The exercise is beneficial for your entire ab area.

Stiff-Legged Deadlift

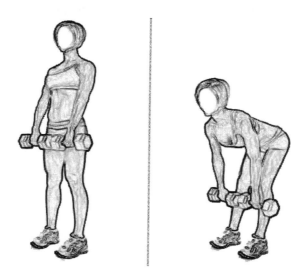

o   Holding a dumbbell in each hand, stand straight. Keep your feet shoulder-width apart and palms facing your legs.

o   Starting from your hips, bend forward and gently lower the dumbbells in front of you until the dumbbells touch the floor.

o   Then go back to the standing position while keeping your back straight.

Close-Hand Pushup

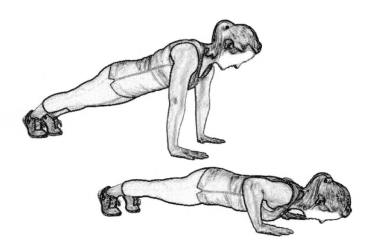

o   The exercise is beneficial for you entire upper body including triceps.

o   Perform push-ups by placing your hands close together. If performing them on your toes is difficult for you then do them on your knees and then gradually work your way toward the toes.

o   If keeping your hands closer is hard for you then keep them further apart when starting.

Conclusion

This exercise book is for those energetic women who want to improve how they are living. The book shows that you don't need advanced fitness machines to lose weight and get fitter. Practice only dumbbells or free hand exercises and feel the difference in days.

Made in the USA
Coppell, TX
14 December 2023

26228807R00035